I0704080

Winning Against
ALLERGIES

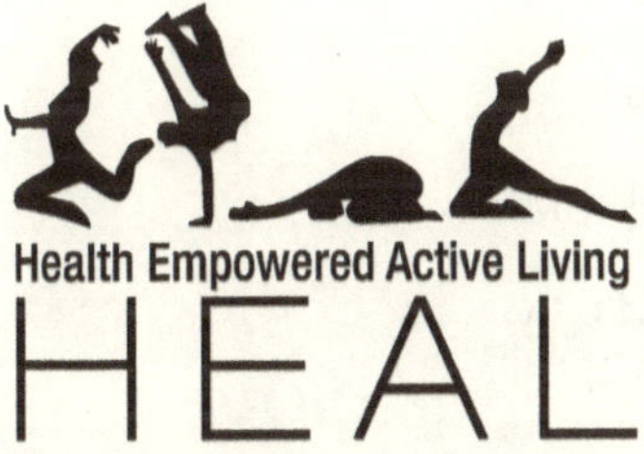

Health Empowered Active Living
HEAL

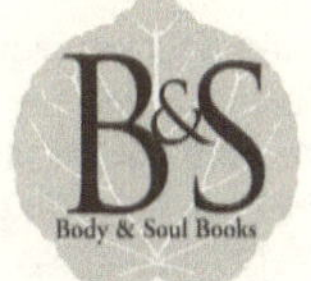

Body & Soul Books

ISBN 978-93-81115-59-6
© Leadstart Publishing Pvt Ltd

Design   Mishta Roy
Layouts   Ajay Shah
Printing   Dhote Offset, Mumbai

Published in India 2011, by
BODY & SOUL BOOKS
an imprint of
LEADSTART PUBLISHING PVT LTD
Trade Centre, Level 1
Bandra Kurla Complex
Bandra (E), Mumbai 400 051, INDIA
T   + 91 22 40700804
F   +91 22 40700800
E   info@leadstartcorp.com
W   www.leadstartcorp.com

US Office
Axis Corp
7845 E Oakbrook Circle
Madison, WI 53717, USA

All rights reserved
No part of this publication may be reproduced, stored in or introduced into a retrieval system, or transmitted, in any form, or by any means (electronic, mechanical, photocopying, recording or otherwise), without the prior permission of the Publisher. Any person who commits an unauthorised act in relation to this publication can be liable to criminal prosecution and civil claims for damages.

Disclaimer *The contents of this book do not purport to replace expert advice or obviate the role of the physician*

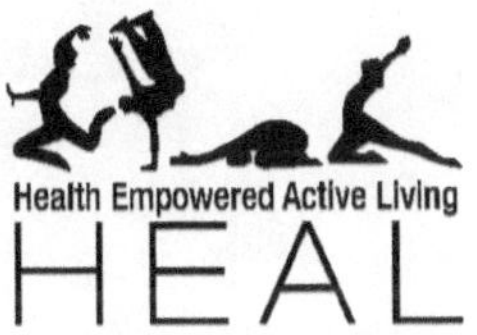

H E A L

ABOUT THE H E A L SERIES

As modern lifestyles move increasingly towards urban and urban-influenced living, our bodies too, face new and mutating challenges to cope with more processed food, less mobility, more time spent indoors in temperature controlled environments, less in green spaces and clean air, more exposure to television, computer, film and telephone screens and less to natural colours, sounds and sunlight. The natural way has become replaced by the artificial way, the instant recourse and quick-fix options.

In all ancient civilizations, stillness and peace were part of the way people lived, in harmony with the earth and nature. Now we have to go looking for it in spas and wellness farms. Stress has become ingrained in human endeavours. We have to consciously de-stress, meditate, do breathing exercises, in order to find equilibrium. What we once accepted as a natural process of fitness and living, is now a search and challenge for health empowerment.

But one thing has not changed – that good health remains the cornerstone of living life to its potential. Only the way in which we seek that elusive grail has changed. And yet, the core truths of health and healing remain the same, based on the five senses: Sight, Smell, Taste, Touch and Hearing. To these five is added one more: Silence – the art of being centred in stillness, where and when mind and being are in harmony.

This series of books has been developed to create holistic health consciousness and education in order to empower strong, active and fulfilled lives. Health remains the foundation on which we build our achievements, both collective and individual. These books are to meant to give laypeople a basic understanding of various ailments and diseases, as well as indicate the solutions available to them. The books do not seek to replace expert advice or the role of the physician.

To be informed is to be empowered. Decision-making and actions flow from knowledge, not general opinion or ignorance. To accept the challenges of our own health in an era of dynamic change all around – that is the ultimate goal.

ॐ

CONTENTS

CONTENTS

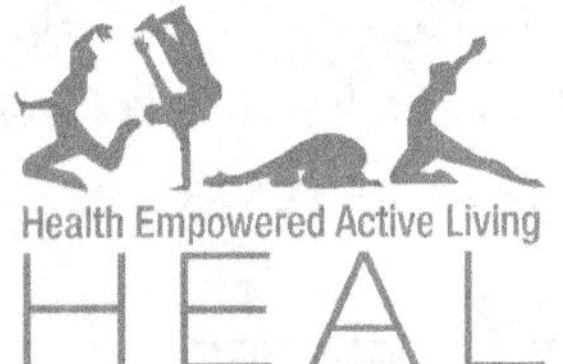
Health Empowered Active Living
HEAL

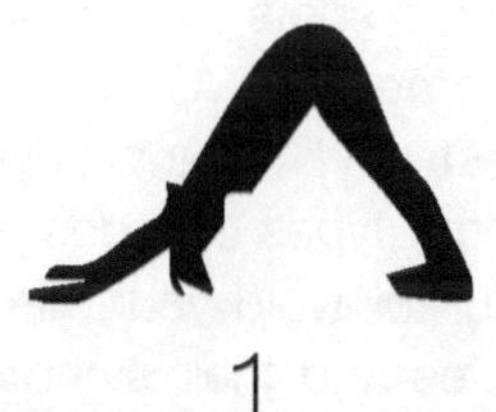

1

UNDERSTANDING ALLERGIES

COMMON ALLERGIES & THEIR SYMPTOMS

If you have these sudden attacks of itchiness, asthma, sneezing, coughing, rashes and red spots all over your body, chances are, you are allergic to something. Common allergies and their symptoms can manifest anytime and anywhere, so if you have allergic reactions to some types of foods, smells, pollen etc, you need to be very careful to avoid your allergy triggers. Note that certain common allergies and their symptoms can cause some serious complications in your body and your general health suffers. To help you understand common allergies and their symptoms, read on.

Common allergies and their symptoms can be broadly categorized into outdoor and indoor allergy triggers. Both types of allergies can make your life really miserable so be aware of the things that could trigger your allergic reactions. For instance, the most common allergies and their symptoms may be caused by different kinds of pollen which comes from trees, weeds, grasses and shrubs.

Technically, pollen is a harmless powdery substance that is emitted into the air by male plants to pollinate female plants. In other words, pollen is necessary to make plants grow and bear fruit. Unfortunately, there are people who are allergic to it. Since pollen is made up of tiny particles and can be inhaled by humans, people who are allergic to it suffer from different forms of allergies and symptoms caused by this. Though it is important for the plants, it is not so for humans.

When inhaled, these tiny particles of powdery substance cause many people to either gasp for breath or start to sneeze.

Inhalation of pollen mostly causes an asthmatic attack or allergic rhinitis in a person. The weather also further contributes to worsen the allergy. Experts are of the opinion that when the weather is moist it further makes it worse. This is because the pollen gets trapped in the moist air and remains in the atmosphere for a longer period causing more attacks. That is why many people who suffer from allergies find that they become worse during cold weather. According to experts, humidity amplifies the allergic reactions as well. Pollen trapped the moisture can stay longer in the air and this cause extended suffering.

While outdoor allergens are seasonal, allergens indoors are present throughout the year. Those people who live cooped up in apartments with no windows and in areas which are highly polluted, will find that they are more prone to allergies. This is because of the continuous presence of molds and mites in such places. The congested air which does not circulate, becomes trapped in the same place, causing people living there to have allergic reactions all the time.

ಉ೦ಚ

FINDING HELP & ALLERGY RELIEF

Allergies are abnormalities we endure. The reactions are physical, yet allergies can affect the emotional state quite perceptably. Since we suffer swellings, aches, and irritations such as running eyes and noses, allergies can make us feel irritated.

Allergens are what cause allergies. Sometimes the substances that cause allergy attacks are toxin. For instance, we may feel the effects after breathing in gas from exhaust pipes on vehicles. We may experience sinus or allergy attacks after breathing in pesticides. Sometimes we are allergic to household chemicals such as cleaners.

Allergies occur also from non-toxic chemicals or substances. We can develop allergies from mould, foods, pollen, and so on. Most allergens that we are exposed to causes allergies, since they build Immunoglobulin E. This antibody causes a histamine reaction, which builds in the tissues of our cells.

Sometimes we are sensitive to medications, toxins and non-toxic substances or chemicals. In these cases, we may experience what appear to be allergic symptoms. We often misinterpret these symptoms as allergies, which find relief once the body recognizes such allergens. Pet dander, milk, mould, pollen, dust, dust mites, proteins, vitamins, medications, etc can cause sensitivity or allergic reactions.

Sensitivity to chemicals can cause watery eyes, running nose, stuffiness and headache. You may feel fatigue. Your digestive system may not work normally. Sometimes you may experience bloating, gas and so on. When sensitivity emerges, most often there is an underlying allergy.

How do allergies start? They can begin from sensitivities to particular particles in the air, substances or chemicals. Even natural growths such as grass, can cause allergies, since fabricated chemicals often contaminate grass. Pet dander can cause a reaction, since unnatural elements attack animal hair.

The immunity system plays a vital part in why allergies start. Our immune system begins to slow its functionalities once we pass thirty. According to medical experts, our immune system, when it begins to slow, can develop various illnesses, including allergies. Respiratory disorders can also start allergies.

Sometimes the pulmonary is obstructed, which starts the conditions known as asthma, emphysema and bronchitis. When the bronchia air is obstructed from its natural flow, serious health hazards do arise.

Doctors consider in their examinations, congenital weakening of the bronchial and pulmonary structure and also irritants that affect the respiratory system. This could include chemicals, pollution in the air and smoke.

Respiratory tract infections are also considered and genetics and predispositions may be evaluated as well. Allergies may start bronchiectasis, in which condition, infection destroys the bronchial mucosa.

If someone has asthma, it is often because the bronchial tree is irritated, which causes broncho constrictions. This narrows the airway due to inflammation. Most times the condition causes mucus to build up and dyspnea. This condition is reversible.

Allergies can cause coughs. When you notice this reaction, you should seek medical help. Mostly, you may find allergy relief, but your doctor may want to monitor your condition, making sure you do not develop bronchitis. Bronchitis occurs from smoke, chemical irritations and air pollution. Recurrence of this condition can lead to chronic coughing.

An allergy is a reaction to something. Sometimes allergies start when we breathe in perfumes that we are sensitive to. To avoid allergic reactions we have to remove ourselves from the triggers. Help and relief are available with your doctor, doctor, over-the-counter medications, herbs, and so on. Allergy relief is available also through self-help programmes.

৪৩

ALLERGIC SYMPTOMS & WHEN TO SEEK MEDICAL HELP

We must know when to seek medical help in case of allergic symptoms. Normally, we never know when we are about to be stricken with an allergy. Common allergic symptoms are running nose, sneezing, watery eyes, itching and hives on the skin. Allergies can strike anyone, anytime and just about anywhere, if allergens are around. Most allergies can be treated easily using over-the-counter or homeopathic medications and even by just avoiding the triggers.

But there are certain allergies which can be life- threatening if not treated immediately. They can even result in death if the symptoms are severe. This is the reason why we should understand the difference between allergies with symptoms that are classified as mild, moderate or severe, and when to seek medical help.

The symptoms which can be termed mild are those which we normally experience like sneezing, watery eyes, itching and nasal congestion. Sometimes there might even be rashes on the skin or hives. Often the symptoms do not spread all over the body and can be termed as very mild. If you find rashes spreading all over your body, then you are in for a more serious problem. These mild symptoms can be treated using nasal decongestants, eye drops, anti-histamines and topical creams for hives and rashes. These do not warrant a visit to a doctor unless they persist for more than two weeks.

Allergic symptoms can be termed moderate to severe if the symptoms spread all over the body and when they threaten the patient's life. Symptoms such as continuous itching and difficulty in breathing, can be termed moderate while severe symptoms include swelling in different parts of the body which can even cause discomfort while swallowing food or breathing problems. Sometimes nausea, diarrhea and vomiting can also occur in severe cases. At times the patient may feel dizzy or disoriented. The moment you find yourself suffering from any of these symptoms, seek immediate medical help. It is important and advisable. These are symptoms of the life- threatening condition called anaphylaxis.

Normally, most allergies that occur in people are mild and can be quite easily treated using over-the- counter prescriptions or home remedies. But having knowledge of severe allergic symptoms will help you to seek immediate medical help if the situation warrants.

Some people choose to take shots to control allergic reactions. Some prefer to induce small amounts of allergens that affect us into our meals to build the immune system's ability to tolerate the allergens. Do not do this at home. Help centres for allergy relief will guide you.

ॐ

COMMON ALLERGY RELIEF TREATMENTS

So you say you have a cold. That sore throat, runny nose, and watery eyes just do not feel good. You have done almost everything you know to do for a common cold. You still do not have any relief.

Perhaps you have an allergy? Did you know that millions of people suffer from some kind of allergy? Even your pets can have some kind of allergy. But luckily, relief is available.

How can I find relief from my allergies? If you feel the allergies are mild, then you may want to test the over-the-counter remedies. Herbs are available to treat allergies also. But if the symptoms persist, the first thing you should do is pay a visit to your doctor. He/She may discourage you from taking over-the-counter remedies. Sometimes doctors will give you Leukortrine blockers. This medicine blocks all chemicals that cause you to have allergies and prevent the recurrent symptoms.

Your doctor may recommend Allegra, Benadryl, Chlor-trimeton, Clarniex, Claritin, Dimetapp or Zyrtec. These medications will give you some relief.

There are also nasal sprays that will help you. Your doctor can help you get started. You should not medicate yourself and cause harm – so check with your family doctor before taking any kind of medication.

What can happen if you are not treated for your allergies? Allergies are not good for anyone, especially if not treated. They can cause many medical problems including asthma, sinus infection or upper lung infection. All these are conditions that have to be treated by a doctor. The best thing to do is go to the doctor in the first place before the condition gets severe.

What can you do to get relief if you have indoor allergies? Cleaning your home can give you some relief. Your pets can have dandruff, causing allergies. Therefore, if you have a pet you may want to inquire from the vet about shampoos to treat dandruff. You can also research the market, since over-the-counter remedies are available. A simple bath often relieves allergic symptoms.

Indoor allergies can irritate the eyes, nose and ears. Look into air purifiers to find allergy relief. The purifiers keep your home free of dust and other particles in the air that causes allergies.

Did you know that various nasal medications can create systematic Rhinitis Medicamentosa? Some medications can cause congestion, these include Aldomet, BuSpar, Cardizem, Comazine, Corgard, Desyrel, Prozac, Procardia, Proventil, Intal and so on.

Other medications can cause a runny nose, and include Capoten, Demulen, Emcyt, Feldene, Lortab ASA, Lozol, Nicorette and Norzine.

Medications that cause bleeding include, Ansaid, BuSpar, Cardizem, Comparzine, Indocin, Moduretic, Orudis and so on. Prozac is a common medication used to treat depression, which can cause bleeding as well.

If you have any symptoms arising from medications you take, speak with your doctor. In fact, when you are prescribed any medications named here, monitor your reactions to help your doctor determine side-effects that may develop from the medications.

Most doctors consider sensitivities to medications before prescribing them, but in some instances unobserved or underlying sensitivities may become apparent only when the reaction occurs.

80CR

ACUPUNCTURE IN ALLERGY RELIEF

If you prefer not to take drugs and looking for some other alternative, Acupuncture may be the answer to your health problems by maintaining balance and harmony after testing to pinpoint the exact allergens that are causing your symptoms. Acupuncture is painless and makes the body strong where it was weak.

Acupuncture uses very fine needles tapped in through tubes. The needles are so small that most people do not even realize they have been inserted into the skin. This method is also used for treating injuries and illnesses caused by drugs.

After acupuncture, you no longer need to avoid what was making you sick. It re-programmes the brain and nervous systems and rebalances your body energy when in contact with the offending allergens.

Although foreign to traditional Western methods of treating allergies, acupuncture, an art which originated in China, is finding widespread acceptance for its pain-free, non-invasive methodology and lasting effects.

ॐॐ

VINEGAR & ALLERGY RELIEF

We have to learn to clean our homes to avoid irritants that cause allergies. Chemicals are all around us and some cleaners we use have harmful chemicals that can kill us if inhaled or digested.

How vinegar works

Vinegar is distilled. It is made of grains and acidity products that come from natural sources. Vinegar has a strong aroma that detracts most people from using the product, yet if you were to clean your home with vinegar, the irritants will stay away also. They too hate the nasty aroma that comes from vinegar!

Most chemicals we use for cleaning have elements that interrupt the respiratory system, bronchia and sinuses. If we are to find allergy relief, we must convert to a new way of living. This means we should only use natural products to clean our homes.

Lysol is a common household cleaning product used by many people. Yet some people suffer severe headaches after using it. This is due to Lysol containing an active ingredient known as dimethylbenzylammonium chloride, which is said to eliminate germs.

The chemicals in Lysol are far less hazardous than other chemicals according to experts. Yet, the chemicals when we are overexposed to them, are toxic. The toxics are linked to birth defects, cancers, and allergy attacks.

One thingis certain, many household cleaning products contain toxins. Anything toxic should surely be worth keeping out of our environment. Most of the air fresheners, soaps, bleaches, shampoos, antiperspirants, hair sprays, cleansers, detergents, paint thinners and so on, are toxic.

Still we have to clean our homes. Instead of using chemicals with harmful toxics, take your cleaning journey to organic reserves.

Vinegar is great for removing stains. Vinegar will keep away irritants. You can also use natural products made by SFI products. Most of these products are safe to use. In fact, thousands of people have tried these products and have given good reports. Go online to check reviews before considering the product. Often, the vendors enable you to make money from selling the products as well. For the most part, you want to think health, so consider the natural, organic options available for allergy relief and a healthy environment.

శుభ

BREATHING LESSONS IN ALLERGY RELIEF

Breathing patterns are very important if you have allergies. When a person cannot breathe, they begin to panic and learning how to control breathing is necessary for everyone. Changing our breathing patterns can be done with little effort. Learning the basic techniques and some practice will help us to take control of breathing.

Breathing comes naturally from birth but as we age, it sometimes needs to be changed to keep us healthy. In order to change our pattern, we have to understand a little bit how breathing techniques work. It is a known fact that practicing new breathing techniques can help prevent attacks and help you to maintain a normal and healthier life.

How inhaling works
As we inhale, our brain sends a message to the diaphragm (that is the muscle separating the heart and lungs from the stomach). When the message gets to the diaphragm, it activates it. The diaphragm will flatten out, letting the lower ribs swing out so that the chest cavity can increase. As the chest cavity increases, air is pulled into the lower lungs.

How exhaling works
When we exhale, the lungs and muscles go back to their normal size. After a pause, the process starts all over again with the brain

sending its message. The normal process of breathing is 14 times a minute or more, depending on how much the person needs it.

Breathing is controlled by the nervous system to run in a self-correcting mode. There are two branches to the self-correcting mode: one is the 'relaxation response', and the other is the 'fight response'.

How the relaxation response works

The relaxation response tells the system to slow down the heart and breathing rate. It works to keep the digestion and elimination going at the normal rate.

How the fight response works

The fight response reacts to the functions that relate to emergencies and exercises. This response awakens and rouses our system to respond to an emergency by pumping adrenaline and making the heart and breathing increase their rate. The increased rate supplies more oxygen to the body. If we are in real danger, the energy is used, if not, it could cause anxiety and hyperventilation.

How breathing fast affects you

With allergies or asthma, we tend to breathe faster without realizing it. Breathing at a faster rate takes more energy but lets us have more oxygen. At the same time, when we breathe out, we lose more much carbon dioxide. If we lose too much carbon dioxide, it can be critical. The hemoglobin that carries the oxygen through the blood to the cells, become sticky and do not let oxygen through.

Learn to slow down your breathing rate to reduce your attacks. There are exercises that can be done to help you to breathe calmly. Continue taking the medications prescribed by your physician before starting to learn new breathing techniques.

How yoga trains you to breathe naturally

Yoga exercises teach you how to practice and learn new breathing techniques. You can join a Yoga group or buy CDs, videos and books about yoga. It is however, advisable to go to an experienced instructor to start yoga as you can injure yourself without proper training.

Studies showed that yoga could reduce allergies by over 60%. Learning and practice is the next step for you and your health. The respiratory system requires care to help you find allergy relief.

ॐॐ

REACTIONS TO ALLERGIES ARE NOTHING TO SNEEZE AT

Most doctors and researchers are still quite confused as to why certain things cause allergies in some people. It is often difficult to pinpoint the exact reason why someone is allergic to a particular thing while the same thing may have no reaction on another person. But dealing with these symptoms can be hard. An allergy can be anything from a sneeze to a running nose, to an anaphylactic shock, which can lead to death.

Doctors are of the opinion that when immunity is low in a person, they are prone to allergies. When the immune system perceives that an alien object is harmful to the body, it gets ready to fight off the intruder and so begins to produce a number of symptoms like hives or rashes on the skin, running nose, watering eyes and sneezing. The moment the alien object leaves the body, the symptoms of allergy also subsides. But there can be many occasions when the symptoms take an extended time to subside.

There are ways to prevent certain allergies. Many people are allergic to dust and so any sweeping or dusting immediately causes reactions. Pollen from flowers are also known to cause allergies. By using a vacuum cleaner which has an inbuilt filter, it is possible to remove dust and dust mites from our surroundings. One can also fit filtering systems in the house as protection from airborne pollens.

Mould and mildew are a major problem for people with allergies and it can be very harmful for the immune system. There are special products to get rid of just mould and mildew and they come as both powders and sprays.

Allergies are often disadvantageous. For example, people who are allergic to hair will find they cannot have a pet dog or cat as the hair from the animal's body can trigger off a series of chain reactions in their body. Pets and odours in your home need to be kept allergen free. Make sure when buying your pet supplies, that they will not add to dust mites and animal allergens.

When buying your laundry supplies to keep the allergens down in the home, be sure to read the labels. You need one for people that are sensitive to allergies. Your laundry detergent should be free from perfume, bleach and any harsh chemicals and used in hot or cold water.

Controlling mould and dust mites can be partly done through humidity control in the home. Dust mites die when humidity is below 50%. Mould lives for humidity so keeping it low kills the mould. dust mites stay alive in your bedding by living off skin shed from your body, so be sure to keep the mattress, box springs and pillows encased with a zipper closing.

Vacuuming the carpet and furniture should be done two or three times a week to help reduce the allergens in the home. A vacuum cleaner with a filter is recommended for the effective removal of allergens from the air. Instead of seeing dust fly from your sweeper as you commonly do with ordinary vacuum cleaners, check out the filtered sweepers. Your vacuum cleaner should include attachments for cleaning those hard-to-get-at spaces and corners and which can be used on furniture. Dust mites are everywhere so be sure to get under you cushions too.

Air filtrations are something every home needs to keep the air clean of all those dust mites flying around. Breathing fresh air is important for people with allergies. When going to buy a filter, be sure to know your room size and get one based for that room or larger. The larger your unit is, the better cleaning job it will do for you. Keep your home environment clean and everyone will be healthier.

Though there are many tests to determine the causes of allergies, the skin prick test is by far the best. This test is best conducted under the supervision of an allergy specialist. What the doctor does is inject each and every item they feel is causing allergy into the patient's body. This helps to narrow down what exactly the causes are.

There are many allergy medications which patients can take so that they can continue with their normal routines. There are also medications which can stop the allergy even before it causes an attack. It is always better to test for allergies before you decide to take any particular medication for it.

శ్రీర

ALLERGIES & FREQUENT URINATION

People know the common effects of allergies: runny nose, sneezing, itchy eyes or hives. However, there can be a number of different ways your body reacts to allergies and range from headaches to gastric problems. frequent urination is a symptom many people do not realize exists. It mostly depends on your allergic trigger and your body's sensitivity to it.

Here are a couple of reasons why allergies and frequent urination could occur.

Medications

Allergies and frequent urination could be tied to the medicines you are taking – many of which have side effects, one being frequent urination. Before you stop taking the medication, visit your doctor and rule out any other causes such as a urinary tract infection. If your medicine is the problem, your doctor will suggest an alternative. It is sometimes frustrating when it takes some time and trial to get the right medication for your individual case. Be patient – it is much better than the alternative of running to the restroom.

Wheat Allergies

Wheat allergies are one of the rarest forms of food allergies, but it does exist. When a person is allergic to wheat, they are allergic to the protein in wheat called gluten. The body sometimes overreacts to the gluten, producing a large number of antibodies and causing an array of symptoms such cramps, loose motions and asthma. Wheat allergies and frequent urination have also been linked. The only way to remedy this condition is to eliminate wheat from your diet. With people becoming more health conscious and offering wheat alternatives, this could pose a problem but paying attention to this detail will pay off.

One way to track if allergies and frequent urination are related, is to keep a food journal. Log everything you eat and drink in a day. You may find that after you have a particular type of food, you are visiting the bathroom more often. This could happen especially with foods and beverages that are acidic such as sodas, coffee and salsa. Such a journal is a big help to your doctor as well in making a final diagnosis.

Allergies and frequent urination could be a problem if it is affecting your work or personal life. There is no real reason why you are experiencing this particular symptom except that your body is having an adverse chemical reaction. If you are suffering from frequent urination consult a doctor because there could be a more serious problem such an enlarged prostate, prostate cancer or a urinary tract infection.

ଓଓ

EXERCISE INDUCED ALLERGIES

Some people have allergic reactions after exercising and it is sometimes responsible for triggering attacks such as asthma.

But isn't exercise supposed to be good for us? How is it possible for exercise to trigger asthmatic attacks?

Good question!

One would think that the only way to promote healthy bones and joints would not trigger asthmatic reactions. However, medical experts believe that this reaction is triggered in some people after working out because the person breathes rapidly during exercise. This causes the airway to dry up and narrow down. Once the person cools down and warm up again, the airways become constricted and hence affect easy breathing.

৯০৫৪

ASTHMA & ALLERGY RELIEF

Allergies can cause you to wake during the night, struggling to breathe. It can lead to suffocation. Allergies affect the chest, throat and breathing. Some problems that emerge from allergies include sneezing, coughing, watery eyes, running nose, aching head, and so on.

Asthma and allergies affect millions of people each year. They cause swelling, leading to shallow breathing. The person breathes heavily and swiftly, gasping for air. The condition awakens them during the night hours, causing them to gag or grasp for air. Breathing being affected, it makes the sufferer feel completely helpless.

Asthma alone can set up as pneumonia and cause the person to grasp for air. Asthma affects the respiratory system, including the bronchial and pulmonary area. It is a disease that affects the lungs and causes inflammation in the airway. The person wheezes, struggles to breathe and so on. Asthma causes flare-ups, coughing, swelling, muscle tightness, mucus build-up, etc.

Some people are born with Asthma, which goes away as they mature. In many instances, the condition turns to allergies. Others, however, continue throughout their lives with asthmatic symptoms. Asthma may include mild symptoms which develop into severe conditions. The condition is, however, life-threatening and Asthma requires ongoing medical observation and treatment.

Allergies affect millions of people each day, yet to find relief, individual studies must take place. We are all different, so we have to find what works best for each of us.

Studies show that yoga is a wonderful healing agent. When we practice yoga, we practice natural breathing. Natural breathing helps to gain control of our respiratory system but beyond that to the entire body and mind. To practice yoga, however, one must first have the will to take control of oneself. If you want relief, yoga is often the answer.

৪৩

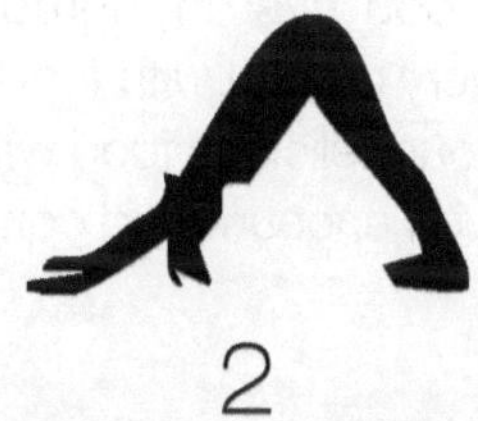

2

FOOD ALLERGIES

FOOD ALLERGY &
HOW TO FIGHT IT

Isn't it annoying when you smell the delicious aroma of a meal only to find that the food has an ingredient to which you are allergic? The bane of every person with food allergies! It is no fun to watch other people devour delicious food which you cannot savour. How many times have you encountered comments like, 'great food isn't it'?

What is food allergy? What causes these annoying symptoms? What is happening inside the body during allergic reactions? Understanding one's condition will better help to accept and overcome the problems.

To start with, food allergy is an unusual reaction to certain types of food allergen. An allergen is the substance or thing that causes the allergic reactions. Exposure to these allergens sets off the alarm in the human immune system which consequently releases antibodies to fight off the invasion of the perceived foreign body (the food allergen). It then causes the symptoms you would see when you are in a state of allergic reaction.

This is just an overview of the whole picture. Looking more closely, allergic reactions undergo two courses of action. The initial course is the release of immunoglobulin E or IgE by the immune system into the bloodstream. IgE is a food-specific antibody and protein that is the body's immune defense against the food allergen.

Following the initial response is the attachment of the IgE to the mast cells. These mast cells are present in body tissues at locations in the body where allergic reactions are common. These locations may include the lungs, skin, nasal and oral cavities, and the gastrointestinal system.

As for the food itself, you may notice that you are not just allergic to just one type of food. There are instances when you may experience an allergic reaction to oyster and then find that you are also allergic to crab and other sea food. This occurrence is what medical professionals call cross-reactivity, wherein an individual can be allergic to closely related or similar types of foods.

The only way to deal with this unfortunate situation is to try to avoid the foods that set off allergic reactions. There is no cure for food allergy but there are medications which can alleviate its symptoms. With the help of a medical health professional, you can be assisted to avoid exposure to food allergens. Nutritionists may teach you alternative ingredients or foods to replace the one to be eliminated from your diet. Also, make it a habit to check food labels for possible ingredients that you may be allergic to and do not hesitate to warn restaurant employees serving you, about your food allergy, in order to prevent any accidents.

Individuals who are highly allergic are advised to wear medical-alert necklaces or bracelets which declare your condition. As for medications, those who are most vulnerable, are also advised to carry with them at all times a self-injectable epinephrine, prescribed by the doctor. This can be of great help during sudden allergic attacks before seeking the assistance of an emergency team.

Other medications are antihistamines, bronchodilators, and corticosteroids. Antihistamines help improve symptoms of rhinitis, hives, rashes, and gastrointestinal problems. Corticosteroids alleviate the severity of inflammations of the skin and in other areas of the body. Bronchodilators are utilized to open up the air passage if it has become inflamed, resulting in breathing difficulties.

To understand more about your food allergies, you must consult your physician. There are also comprehensive books that have complete information about food allergies and how to fight them.

ॐ

FOOD ALLERGIES & DIMINISHED APPETITE

Since most people like to eat, it can be depressing to learn they have developed food allergies. No matter how good a particular dish may taste, it is not worth the potential swelling, itching and potential for death, to consume a food product knowing it can ignite a reaction. While different people may suffer food allergies from different foods, some of the most common are peanuts and shell fish. Most will learn of an allergy the first time they are exposed to it, but allergies can often develop later in life and come as a surprise.

When a person consumes a particular food and has an allergic reaction, their best plan is to eliminate that item from their diet. The symptoms of food allergies are very similar to other types of allergies and may include a runny nose, watering eyes, skin rash and hives. Other reactions can include headache due to sinus infections and pain in the ears as well as diminished hearing.

In some individuals, food allergies can also cause an anaphylactic reaction which causes a sudden lowering of blood pressure as well as difficulty in breathing. In the most severe cases, it can cause death.

Finding the cause before it kills

In most cases, the cause of food allergies are easy to determine by maintaining a food diary and recording any adverse reactions related to specific foods. Once the list has been narrowed down, any food that causes an allergic reaction should be avoided. To pinpoint the exact cause of food allergies, your doctor may recommend the skin prick test before they cause serious health problems.

Foods contain a multitude of ingredients and it could simply be one of the ingredients that cause food allergy. If the product can be found without that specific ingredient, it will not continue to be a problem. Reading labels may seem time consuming and boring but will identify such ingredients before they cause you health issues. When eating out at restaurants it is not always possible to identity all ingredients but make sure you inform the waiter taking your order.

Children are the most common sufferers from food allergies as they normally do not remember or regard what causes allergies in them and consume any food. If a child has an allergic reaction, it is best to get help quickly so that the condition does not worsen. A child who is prone to food allergies should wear a medical-alert bracelet so that they can be identified and treated if they accidentally consume foods that can cause allergies.

ॐ॑

COMMON FOOD ALLERGIES & HOW TO TREAT THEM

Common food allergies are some of the most common types of allergies that exist. When you initially eat a food, you may not know you are allergic to it. Minor symptoms of common food allergies usually result in swelling and tingling of the lips, tongue and mouth. More severe allergies include trouble breathing, swelling of the throat, vomiting and fainting. These conditions require immediate attention as they can cause fatalities. The common term for this is anaphylaxis shock. People with common food allergies can also suffer from upset stomachs, skin rashes or itchy, swollen eyes. There is no standard symptom for common food allergies so it is important to note all the reactions you have.

The good thing about common food allergies is that if you stay away from these foods, the allergies will not be a problem. There have been eight foods that are widely associated with common food allergies.

- ✓ Milk
- ✓ Eggs
- ✓ Peanuts
- ✓ Tree nuts
- ✓ Fish
- ✓ Shellfish
- ✓ Soy
- ✓ Wheat

About 90 percent of common food allergies can be related to these eight foods. In the USA, for instance, companies and restaurants are required by law to state if any of these foods are present.

Reading labels and all warnings on food is important. If you have a peanut allergy but do not realize that a certain snack has peanuts, you could end up suffering a severe reaction. Read the label.

If you think you have a food allergy or notice that after you eat a certain thing, you do not feel well, you may want to check with your doctor to see if you have any allergies. There are ways your doctor or an allergist can check for common food allergies. Such tests include a blood test, skin test and a careful description of what you have eaten. It is smart to keep a journal of foods and write down whenever you have a reaction. This way doctors can use this when deciphering the information and will be able to tell if you have a common food allergy.

If you do have common food allergies, let your doctor know on every visit about this allergy. There are some medications that you might not be able to take because you might have a reaction to them.

ॐकर

WHAT YOUR DOCTORS KNOW ABOUT DIAIRY ALLERGENS

Dairy allergies are not fun to deal with. Those with this allergy can testify to the pain and general inconvenience dairy allergies cause. Symptoms of dairy allergies range from moderate to severe with some of the more common symptoms being loose bowels, vomiting and skin rash. People with asthma may begin to wheeze after having a dairy product (products containing milk).

What are dairy allergies?

Dairy allergies occur when the body has an adverse reaction to a protein found in these products. It is actually one of the most common food allergies. Babies who suffer from dairy allergies often grow out of the allergy once they reach three years of age. However, parents still need to be careful and keep a constant vigil over children and their reaction to foods.

Treatment of dairy allergies

Unfortunately for dairy allergy sufferers, the only way to avoid dairy allergies is by avoiding the products. There are no special pills to make the body less reactive. People should avoid milk, butter, cheese and all types of cream. Read the nutritional label and check for anything that could be harmful. There are other items that state the product uses dairy milk: whey, casein, lactic acid and sodium lactate.

If one does ingest a dairy product, there are ways to combat the allergic reaction. Sometimes an Epinephrine pen is used if the allergy is severe and needs immediate attention. Otherwise an antihistamine, more commonly known as Benedryl, could be prescribed to alleviate the allergic reaction.

Alternatives to milk

There are many replacements available to people suffering from dairy allergies. You can find rice milk, soy milk, almond milk and other variations in the supermarket. However, these types of milk are not suitable for a child's nutrition. Get a doctor's recommendation on how to get calcium and other nutrients you are missing out on. Children need extra attention to get the proper nutrition. Look for juices, drinks with added calcium and other products that could help.

Difference between allergies and lactose intolerance

Dairy allergies should not be confused with being lactose intolerant. These are two different problems. If someone suffers from dairy allergies, the body is having an adverse chemical reaction to the protein found in milk products. In a lactose intolerant person, the body cannot process the sugar found in milk because of the absence of lactase. This is a non-allergy reaction. People who are lactose intolerant will also have different symptoms, which are mostly intestinal related: flatulence, stomach cramps, bloating and loose bowels.

ೞಯಲ

COMMON PEANUT ALLERGIES CAN CAUSE FATAL REACTIONS

What are peanut allergies?

Peanut allergies occur when the body has an adverse reaction to peanuts or peanut-containing products. The person's immune system tries to fight off the peanut as it does not recognize it as a substance that is not harmful. The scary thing about peanut allergies is that it is the most common cause of life-threatening allergic reactions. This is a very serious and dangerous allergy and should be treated carefully. Those who suffer from peanut allergies need to be vigilant about the foods they eat.

Symptoms of peanut allergies

Symptoms range from moderate to severe, but either way, they should be treated immediately. A person can suffer from itching, swelling, nausea or abdominal cramps. However, it can get worse than that. Many who have peanut allergies have shortness of breath, wheezing and can lose consciousness (anaphylaxis). One can also develop hives. Usually, symptoms occur within a few minutes of exposure to peanuts, but there have been cases when it took hours. A person suffering from the most serious symptoms, anaphylaxis, requires immediate attention. He/She will have difficulty breathing, the blood pressure will drop and seizures could result.

Foods to avoid

There are many foods that are made with peanuts or cooked in peanut oil. as peanut allergies are so severe that labels now have to state if a product contains nuts, even if there are not any nuts readily seen in the food. Obvious foods to avoid are peanut butter, granola bars, cookies and other types of nuts and energy bars. But take a closer look at some of the other foods a person who has peanut allergies might come into contact with. There are some sauces and salad dressings that are made from crushed nuts. Many baked goods have nuts in them, including cookies, cakes, marzipan. Check potato chips or salty food packages to see if the food was made using peanut oil.

Treatment of peanut allergies

Depending on the severity of the symptoms, a person can have either an antihistamine (Benadryl) or an emergency injection of epinephrine. Those who know they suffer severely from peanut allergy, should carry epinephrine with them at all times. But the only way to not suffer from peanut allergies is to avoid peanuts and all the potential harmful foods as well. If a person thinks they suffer from a peanut allergy, they should see a doctor or allergist who can perform a battery of tests to tell what specific substances a person is allergic to, including peanut allergy.

ഇരു

TREATING FRUIT ALLERGIES

Fruits are very important in a diet as they supply many of the vitamins, minerals and fibre that the body needs to maintain health and strength. But some people find that fruits cause allergic reactions in their bodies. These allergic reactions can be easily recognized and it is always quite easy to say which fruit a person is allergic to. So once the fruit is identified as causing an allergy, it is best to avoid that fruit.

Oral allergy syndrome is very common to fruit allergies as consuming certain fruits cause swellings in the tongue, mouth, lips and throat etc. The moment the fruit comes into contact with the mouth or lips, they begin to burn or swell.

This syndrome is not restricted to fruits alone but also pertains to vegetables. This is caused by the chemical reactions which take place between the pollens and proteins. It is a common phenomenon that people who have fruit allergies are also allergic to pollens. Only when fruits and vegetables are eaten fresh, do they cause allergies in people and not when they are cooked. This is because the pollens and proteins which are present get destroyed when cooked.

Some of the other symptoms which fruit allergies cause are skin irritations, redness and rashes or hives. Sometimes, blood pressure can also drop drastically cutting off oxygen supply to the brain. The mouth, throat and airways begin to swell, restricting air supply to the lungs and this leaves the person gasping for breath which in turn leads to suffocation and death.

Only certain classes of fruits tend to cause allergies. For instance, if one is allergic to rag weed, then when one eats fruits like bananas and melons like cantaloupe and honeydew, it will cause allergic reactions.

In the case of Birch tree allergy, certain fruits like apples, pears, cherries, kiwi and stone fruits are more likely to cause reactions. Certain other fruits like lemons, oranges limes and grapefruit, which belong to the citrus variety, can commonly be the cause of allergies. This is mainly due to the acidic nature of the citrus fruits.

The best way to avoid fruit allergies is not to eat those fruits so that all that rashes, swelling and skin irritations can be avoided. There are people who have become resistant to fruit allergies because of the allergy injections which they have taken. There is, however, another option – which is to have the fruits cooked to avoid allergic reactions in your body.

ॐ

HOW TO LIVE WITH WHEAT ALLERGIES

It is quite common to find children suffering from food allergies. The symptoms can also vary from mild to moderate to severe. Wheat is one of the top eight foods which cause allergies. Most of the food that is available contains wheat as an ingredient in one form or the other. Normally, children are the main sufferers of wheat allergies though they soon outgrow the condition. However, adults suffer from wheat allergies too.

The time taken for wheat allergy to show up after the food is eaten, is normally anywhere between a few minutes to a few hours, and the symptoms also can be mild or severe. Anaphylaxis is a life-threatening allergic symptom which needs immediate medical help. Common symptoms of wheat allergy include nasal congestion, swelling of the airway and inflammation, irritations on the skin or hives, or even nausea, vomiting and diarrhea. When the symptoms are severe, the person can experience shock, dizziness, rapid pulse and constriction of the airway. Anyone suffering from these symptoms requires immediate medical help.

If you are suffering from wheat allergies, the best thing to do is to avoid all wheat products in your diet. This will reduce your chances of getting an allergic reaction. The more the reactions, the more severe the allergy is, and therefore it is advisable to see your doctor immediately even if you experience mild symptoms. Your doctor will then carry out a series of tests to find out if wheat was really the culprit. You too will find it easier to avoid wheat products from your diet as most manufacturers make it a point to list it on their food packages.

If you have a severe wheat allergy reaction, your doctor may advise you to take what is called the Epipen treatment. In this treatment, which is done as an emergency measure for wheat allergies, an injection is given. You can also wear a bracelet which alerts people about your wheat allergy problems. Wheat allergy sufferers are normally told to avoid all wheat products in their diets and to take antihistamines if they are stricken by the allergy.

ॐ

A SURVIVAL GUIDE TO OVERCOMING & RECOVERING FROM FOOD ALLERGY

Everyone loves variety in food – however, for some people, certain food items cause allergic reactions and they need to avoid eating those food items. What is food allergy? It is the immunologic effect that is caused by the existence of food proteins.

A simple search on the internet, will give you a list of books and materials that detail food allergy. One such book is, *5 Years without Food: The Food Allergy Survival Guide: How to Overcome Your Food Allergies and Recover Good Healthy*. An interesting book, it explains what food allergy is and what causes them. But just because you are allergic towards a certain food does not mean you have to forfeit the nutrients that you would have got. You also gain an understanding of the food that can be taken as supplements or alternatives. The book also explains a few treatments related to food allergy.

Here is a list which will benefit readers who are prone to food allergy. In general, food such as shellfish, fish, soya, eggs, peanuts, tree nuts may create allergy in adults. Milk, eggs, peanuts are known to create allergies in children. It is always a good idea to be knowledgeable about the food you are allergic to.

Key To Food Items & Allergies
Allergic to eggs
Those who are allergic towards egg are said to be hypersensitive

towards nutritional substances derived from yolk or egg white (albumin, globulin), such as eggnog. This may result in overreaction in the immune system.

It is advisable to stay away from food items made with egg but you need not worry about not eating egg as many substitutes for egg are available in the market today, including potato starch, tapioca, etc., and you may use them without any trouble. You can even use apple sauce as an alternative to egg.

Allergic to tree nuts

Hypersensitivity towards tree nuts is called tree nut allergy. Don't confuse tree nuts with peanut allergy. They are different. Dry fruits are tree nuts, whereas peanuts are legumes. Children are more prone to nut allergies than are adults.

You can use soy nuts as an alternative to tree nuts. However, to clarify a point, soy nut goes through a soaking process and is then baked, to get the crispy soy nut.

Allergic to milk substances

Are you allergic towards proteins that are present in cow's milk? If so, you can use rice milk or soy milk as substitutes to cow's milk. This way you get the nutrients that would normally have come from cow's milk.

Allergic to seafood

This allergy is caused by the intake of food items such as scaly fish, crustaceans or shellfish. The best way is to stay away from sea food. If you use a lot of canned food items, ensure that they are not made with seafood ingredients.

Be picky about the food items you eat. This may help you surmount the allergic reaction. Certain allergies can be cured in a short period of time; however, certain food allergies cannot really be treated in an entire lifespan.

ఐంౘ

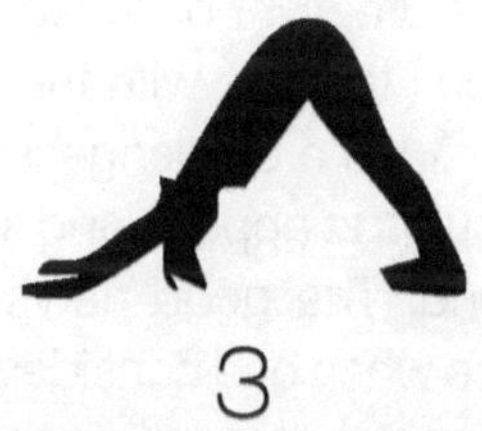

3

MOULD ALLERGIES

UNDERSTANDING & PREVENTING MOULD ALLERGIES

Allergies are common ailments and the substances that people are allergic to varies greatly. For those who suffer from mould allergies, it is often difficult to cope with the symptoms. The reason that mould allergies are such a challenge is because there is not a particular season for moulds to appear, and some people experience symptoms all year round. The good news is that these types of allergies are relatively rare when one considers the varieties of moulds we are exposed to every day. It is also possible to effectively treat mould allergy, so that one does not have to suffer unnecessarily with the sniffling and sneezing that arise from exposure to the dreaded moulds.

Symptoms

Mould allergy symptoms are similar to those of other allergies and include nasal congestion, runny nose, watery eyes, and a skin rash. If you experience any of these while raking leaves or mowing grass, you could be suffering from mould allergy. Likewise, if you notice these symptoms when you enter a musty or moist area, mould may indeed be the culprit. To determine if your allergy is really caused by mould spores, you can have an allergy test done. There are two types of tests: a skin test or a blood sample. Either test will give your doctor a good idea about the substances that you are allergic to so that he can treat you effectively.

Treatment & Prevention

Treatment for any allergy generally includes over-the-counter medications like decongestants or antihistamines. For more severe symptoms, your doctor may prescribe stronger doses. You can also opt for steroidal nasal sprays to keep nasal passages clear, or inhaled medications if you suffer from asthma. Many of these medications are safe to take over a longer period of time, making them good options for mould allergy sufferers who might experience symptoms year round.

Another good way of reducing symptoms is by prevention. This usually entails avoidance of the allergy triggers – which in this case would be mould spores. Prevention of mould allergies would include avoiding food that has a greater chance of harbouring mould, like cheese and mushrooms, or staying away from damp areas like basements. It is also a good idea to change your furnace filter frequently to prevent mould developing. With a combination of prevention and treatment, it is possible to keep your mold allergy symptoms at bay.

৪৩৫

CONSIDER FLUCONAZOLE FOR MOULD ALLERGIES

Allergies that never go away might be a sign of a bigger problem or caused by a substance that has not been explored yet. If the sneezing does not stop and the runny nose continues, perhaps it is not the pollen in the air. You may want to look into mould, which can be a dangerous substance, not just an annoyance. To help with the allergies, a doctor might prescribe Fluconazole, also known as Diflucan.

What is mould allergy?

Let's start with defining mould allergy. These occur when microscopic fungal spores cause allergies when inhaled. The spores are so tiny that they get past the nasal defenses and into the lungs. Mould can be found anywhere in the home. However, the places where mould is more common, are in damp basements, closets and bathrooms. Anywhere where there is moisture, there is the possibility of mould. It does not have to be just inside the home, mould can grow in the garden or yard. So if you are having constant allergy problems, you may want to check if there is mould. Talk to a doctor about the possibility of getting Fluconazole for mould allergies.

Symptoms of mould allergies

Mould allergy symptoms might be difficult to distinguish as they are so like other common allergies. You have to deal with sneezing, runny nose, coughing and post-nasal drip. There is no simple way to tell if you have a mould allergy. A doctor will need to swab your nose and send it to a lab to be tested for mould. Lab tests will be able to tell what type of mould is causing your allergies.

Treatment of mould allergies

There are a few ways to deal with mould allergies. The first step is to remove mould from your home. It is the only way mould allergies are going to ever end. In the meantime, discuss with your doctor medications such as Fluconazole – it comes in both pill and liquid forms. Fluconazole deals with many different problems in the fungi family, which is why it is so effective in the case of mould allergies.

There may be side effects to the drug, so check with your doctor. Side effects to Fluconazole could include nausea, diarrhea and loss of appetite. Those taking medications for diabetes, insomnia or high blood pressure, should avoid Fluconazole for their mould allergies. There could be adverse reactions to other medications you are taking and the best way forward is to discuss this with your doctor and not try to do it yourself.

ৡৎ

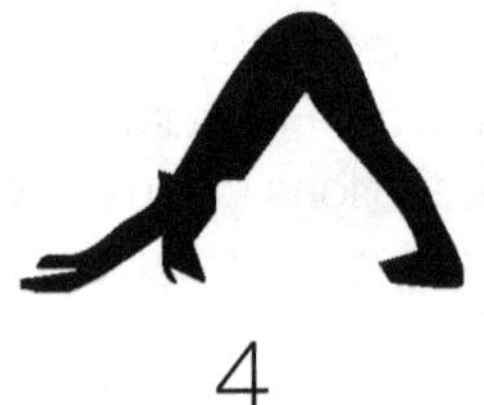

4

SKIN ALLERGIES

WITH ALLERGIES THE DEGREE OF SKIN RASH CAN VARY

Allergic reactions come in many forms. There is the sneezing with the itchy, watery eyes. Others may have trouble breathing when their asthma is triggered by a substance in the air. Skin rashes are common when it comes to allergic reactions. They result from all sorts of triggers, from food to clothing to laundry detergent. Even when going for a stroll in the park, you can walk into something that will give you an allergic skin rash. The key is knowing the differences and taking care of the problem as soon as it happens.

There are different skin rashes that occur from allergies.

Atopic Dermatitis

Another name for this is Eczema. This allergic skin rash has certain characteristics such as dry, itchy skin. It can be aggravated by clothing, laundry detergent, soaps or stress. Often, it is found in families that have a history of asthma or hay fever. The main way to treat Eczema is through proper skin care. Avoid soaps with scents or creams in them. Avoid certain clothing such as wool that can aggravate it. Use warm water when bathing and avoid body lotions with extra ingredients.

Contact Dermatitis

This is a skin rash that is caused by coming into contact with a substance that causes rash. Another way to get Contact Dermatitis is by doing something that irritates the skin. Contact dermatitis most commonly happens when a person comes into contact with poison ivy, poison oak or fake jewellery, to name a few, but these are not the only things that can cause it. Contact Dermatitis only affects the skin where it has been touched. Treatments are usually in the form of topical creams or lotions.

Allergic drug rash

Allergic skin rashes can be caused by reaction to medication. Unfortunately, there is no specific way to test that the skin rash is from an allergy to a particular medicine. The doctor might recommend the patient stop taking the drugs to see if the rash continues.

Hives

Anyone who has had hives knows that this is a terrible allergy. It is a skin rash that can happen on any part of the body. Hives can be caused by other means and not just as an allergic reaction. Hives can be induced by stress or external factors. There is no medicine or cream for hives. The itchy, red bumps need to just take their course.

Not all skin rashes are allergies. Rashes can be caused by other medical conditions. Never self-diagnose. Always go to a doctor or a dermatologist to learn the nature of the skin rash. If it does turn out to be an allergic skin rash, visit an allergist and run tests to find out what you are allergic to. This way you can avoid those substances and stop feeling miserable and itchy.

৪০৫

SKIN ALLERGIES ACCOUNT FOR MOST COMPLAINTS

Skin Allergies are different for every person. They can appear in a confined area or over their entire body. There are even cases when a person has allergic reactions on their hands and feet, making it difficult to do everyday tasks. A skin allergy is called Contact Dermatitis. The skin has a chemical reaction to the substance it has come into contact with. In these cases, one has to physically touch it to get the allergy. Some of the culprits may surprise you.

Testing for skin allergies

One way to find out what causes skin allergies is by playing a guessing game. However, there are no winners in this one. You could test products on your skin to see if have a reaction. But there is an easier way. Doctors do patch testing when they take a small piece of skin (this doesn't hurt) and then put each patch of skin into contact with common allergens. They watch for any reactions.

Here are some of the most common causes of skin allergies.

Nickel & gold

These metals are usually found in jewellery. Nickel is found in clasps or buttons. Gold is more common. Many items are made or plated with gold. If you have an allergy to either of these metals, a rash will break out where the metal has touched your skin. Many people tend to have skin reactions to costume jewellery.

Balsam of Peru

This fragrance is found in many lotions and perfumes. Another name for it is *Myroxylon Pereirae*. If this is the culprit for your skin allergy, check the ingredients in perfumes and lotions you use to see if this is present.

Neomycin Sulfate

This substance is commonly found in first aid creams and ointments. Unfortunately, a doctor might prescribe a topical cream for a previous skin rash, only to discover that the patient also has skin allergies to this substance too. It is also found in cosmetics, soap and pet food.

Bacitracin

This is a topical antibiotic. Some people use it on cuts or burns.

Cobalt chloride

This is a real problem for some people because it is normally found in antiperspirants. However, there are other places cobalt chloride shows up, such as hair dye and plated items such as buttons, snaps and tools.

Quaternium 15

This is a preservative found in many products that women tend to use. It can be found in self-tanners, shampoo, nail polish and sunscreen. Try to find products that do not use this if you have skin allergies to Quaternium 15.

൞

TATTOO ALLERGIES –
AN UNCOMMON BUT
REAL PROBLEM

Tattoos are a popular trend. However, with the onset of the tattoo craze, a problem has emerged – tattoo allergies.

The ink in the artwork contains ingredients that cause the tattoo allergies. The most common allergen is found in red and yellow inks. The problem with tattoo ink is that it is unregulated. Almost anything can be used to create the pigments. Some of the more common ingredients include nickel, mercury (although less and less), cobalt and cadmium.

Signs of the allergy include itchiness around and on the tattoo, raised bumps, redness, irritation or hives. Worse case scenarios include formation of puss and oozing around the tattoo and sores. When this occurs, the person should see a doctor immediately. Usually, a steroid will be given at the site of the problem that will eliminate the allergy.

Just because you get a tattoo and do not have a reaction a week later does not mean you are immune. Tattoo allergies sometimes do not show up right away. There have been cases where the effects appear years later. Usually in such cases, there is something that triggers the reaction, such as another tattoo (creating more exposure), change in the weather or even an illness. The treatment in these cases is the same.

If the allergy is severe, the ink can be removed by a doctor, using a laser. If the allergy is mild and you just suffer from occasional itching or swelling, over-the-counter anti-inflammatory and anti-histamine creams should help. If you ever notice that during the summer months, your tattoo gets itchy or a little red, this could be due to a tattoo allergy. Most people who do have this moderate reaction tend to just deal with the problem with anti-histamine creams.

Unfortunately, there is no way of knowing you are going to have tattoo allergies. There are no tests that can be done beforehand. You can't have a small piece of skin that is out of the way tested because of the length of time some tattoo allergies take to appear. The only time people discover they have a tattoo allergy is after the tattoo is already on the body.

Take into careful consideration what tattoo artists tells you about cleaning your tattoo. This prevents any immediate reactions your body may have and is also an easier way to watch for signs of an allergic reaction. Keep in mind tattoo allergies are rare, so don't shy away from them if you really want to get one.

৪৩

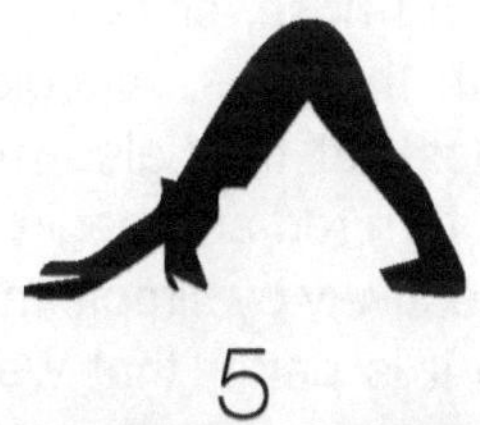

5

EYES & NOSE ALLERGIES

CAUSES & TREATMENT OF
EYE ALLERGIES

When we think of allergies, we normally refer to only symptoms like itching, running nose, sneezing and hives. We rarely associate allergies with the eyes. Allergies not only affect the sinus and nasal cavities but they also make the eyes start to itch, make them swell, turn red and begin to water. Eye allergies can also be treated effectively by simple medications. Prevention is better than cure so it is better that we learn how to protect ourselves from eye allergies first. We should know why they occur and how to treat them.

Our eyes are important organs which are continuously exposed to the external world while we are awake. Because of continuous exposure, the eyes are more susceptible to allergens attacking them and that is why more people get affected easily. Unlike the nose and its passageway, where there are tiny hairs called cilia, which help to filter all harmful bacteria, the eyes do not have such in-built protection and are more prone to being attacked by harmful bacteria.

If you are someone who is already suffering from allergies of any kind, then you can be sure that you will also suffer from eye allergies. So if you have the sneezes due to pollens, then you can be sure that you will also have eye allergies. If you have a family history of allergies or have Atrophic Dermatitis, you are sure to suffer from eye allergies. But do not get disheartened, there are various treatments available that can be used to treat eye allergies.

The best way you can avoid eye allergies is through prevention. If you are aware of what to avoid, then you can take steps to avoid contact and will therefore not be susceptible to it. If you feel that your hands have come into contact with a known allergen, then make sure that you avoid rubbing or touching your eyes with those hands. Many people tend to rub their eyes, not realizing that it is one of the main causes for allergies. If you still feel that despite all precautions, you still seem to have itching and watery eyes, then it is advisable to take medications. These medications can be bought over-the-counter or you can get your doctor to prescribe them for you. They are mainly eye drops which have to be applied a couple of times a day.

It is difficult to cope with eye allergies as they are very uncomfortable and irritating, so it is best that you talk to your doctor to find ways of reducing allergy symptoms.

ഇര

NASAL ALLERGIES

If you are prone to continuous sneezing, then blame it on your genetics and your body's lack of immunity. Allergic rhinitis or nasal allergy is bound to occur in a person if they are exposed to allergens, pollution, cigarette smoke or happen to have a low weight at birth.

Doctors are puzzled as to why some people are allergic to certain substances while others are not, but one thing they are sure about is that your body does indeed respond to these allergens. Your body's immune system has been programmed in such a way as to react whenever a foreign body gets into the nose and this triggers a series of reactions in the body when the immune system begins its fight to repel the substance. During this process, a chemical substance called histamine is released. This is why your eyes begin to water and your nose starts running. At times, more severe problems like wheezing and breathing difficulty, occur.

Often, it is allergens which are present in the atmosphere that are the causes of nasal allergies, though these allergens can come from different sources. One of the main causes of nasal allergies is pollens and their concentration can vary according to the place. Some pollen, like Rag Weed, can travel far and wide, so even if you live in a city, you may still be affected by it. Flowering trees, plants, grass and bushes also release a number of pollen grains into the air causing nasal allergies.

Though dust can cause you to sneeze, it may not cause nasal allergy. But dust mites, which are tiny microscopic organisms which can be found in mattresses, carpets and furniture, do cause nasal allergy. You will know for sure that it is the dust mites which are actually causing you to sneeze when in the winter months the pollens in the air are at a minimal but you still find yourself sneezing endlessly.

Another serious allergic problem is caused by animal dander. Dander comes from pets like dogs and cats who easily settle on carpets and furniture and cause sneezing problems even after you have got rid of your pets. The only way you can get rid of dander once and for all is to get the carpet and upholstery in your home vacuumed and shampooed thoroughly.

You will know that you are having a nasal allergy the moment your nose starts to twitch and you begin sneezing for no reason. It is the body's way of trying to get rid of the allergen. The nose then starts to run and this is how the body's mechanism tries to wash out the allergen. A little later, say after a few hours, you will find that you now having a stuffy nose and have become extremely sensitive to other irritants. You will have to endure this for the duration it takes the body to clear the allergen. Some people can develop more serious problems like asthma or sinus infections.

৅ে

CHRONIC OBSTRUCTIVE PULMONARY DISEASE & ALLERGY RELIEF

Chronic Obstructive Pulmonary Disease (COPD), causes asthma attacks, as well as allergic outbreaks. By definition, COPD is a cluster of disease that stems from unrelenting obstruction of the bronchial air flow. The condition can cause one to suffer chronic bronchitis, bronchiectasis, asthma and emphysema. Smoking is the leading cause of these conditions, yet other irritants in our environment can cause the conditions to emerge also.

When one is battling disease, one needs frequent follow-up visits to the doctor. The symptoms are all important. Inform your doctor as much as you can about your condition. This will help him/her find the treatment that works for you and monitor the effects of medication.

How emphysema affects you

Emphysema is one of the worst conditions related to allergies that one can endure. Emphysema causes a stimulation to affect your breathing pattern, which is when PO-2 commonly decreases (ie. low PCO-2). To find allergy relief, one has to avoid irritants, which in this case is smoke. One will have to stay away from areas where people smoke and avoid smoking tobacco oneself.

What are the possibilities in etiology?

If you are diagnosed with asthma, emphysema or bronchial conditions, your congenital can weaken. The respiratory system is irritated, usually from chemical irritants, polluted air, or smoke. The condition leads to respiratory tract infections. Your doctor will need to monitor this condition on a regular basis.

What symptoms are related to these conditions?

If you suffer from these conditions, you should notice coughing, dyspnea, and usage of accessory muscles, crackles, wheezing, exertional dyspnea and barrel chest. Sputum production is observable when emphysema is present. Asthma or bronchial infections can present anxiousness, anemia, hemoprysis, weight loss, orthopnea, diaphoresis, finger clubbing, malaise, and so on.

If you have common allergies you should avoid irritants in the environment, home, work and so on. Your condition could develop into chronic pulmonary systems in later years. Some of the irritants to avoid include pollen, pet dander, dust mites, dust, and smoke, harsh chemicals, mold, mildew and so on.

Other irritants made of latex can affect you also. Bananas, cherries, apricots, nuts, chestnuts, kiwi, nectarines, celery, are all products that come from latex. Pineapple, plums, melons, potatoes, avocados, tomatoes, peaches, and grapes come from latex trees and shrubs.

How can I fight COPD & allergies?

If you are subject to these conditions, speak with your doctor immediately and follow instructions implicitly.

You will need a healthy diet that provides you with plenty of Vitamin C, proteins, and if possible, nitrogen. You should increase the intake of fluids to about 3,000 milligrams daily.

In addition, you should keep your weight down. We can all benefit from exercise. Set up a schedule that works for you and exercise often. Exercise will help you maintain your weight and reduce your risk of disease.

Sometimes you have to move from your environment when allergies, asthma or other related conditions could affect you. Talk to your doctor. While some people benefit from a warm climate others prefer to move to areas where pollutants in the air are less severe.

Allergy relief can be found in yoga.

More about asthma

Studies show that children are most affected by asthma, and miss many school days because of this condition. Asthma claims more than 100,000 lives annually.

At one time experts believed that environmental irritants were responsible for asthma attacks. New studies in areas where irritants have declined, still show that asthma continues to increase, taking lives.

Some of the evidence found in these studies pointed to medications prescribed to treat allergies and asthma. It is advisable to use yoga and other healthy activities in our daily living in order to avoid side-effects from allergy-based drugs. According to those who study yoga, relief is possible through regular practice. According to recent scientific reports, more people who practiced yoga, found relief, than those who took medications to treat asthma and allergies.

ॐ

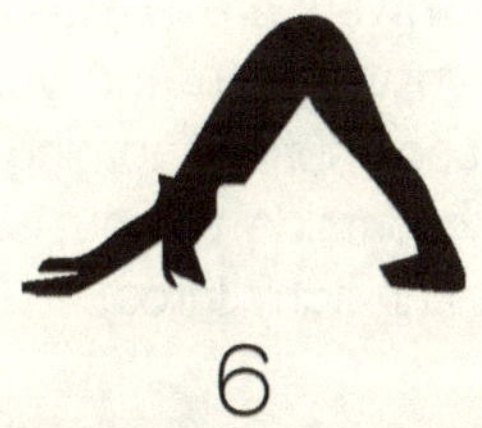

6

ENVIRONMENTAL ALLERGIES

HOW TO COPE WITH SEASONAL ALLERGIES

Anyone who suffers from seasonal allergies knows how daunting spring can be. The flowers are in bloom, the birds are coming back from their southern vacation and you can't stop sneezing! There is nothing like a cool, spring morning when the pollen count is so high, you can't go outside without suffering from sneezing, itching, watery eyes and an itchy throat.

The routine is the same every year and the medicine cabinet is filled with anti-allergy medication. There are those who suffer differently from seasonal allergies. While the common symptoms affect many people, seasonal allergies are worst in people who also suffer from asthma and allergic rhinitis. Seasonal allergies aren't just an inconvenience anymore, but have become a medical problem. People are hospitalized every year from this.

But there are ways to make the seasonal changes easier. Seasonal allergy sufferers do not have to be discouraged every time a new season starts. There are ways to prevent seasonal allergies and tricks to make the allergy season more bearable.

Eating essential fatty acids
Studies show that essential fatty acids and flax seed help reduce allergic reactions in many people. Increase your daily dose of these essential fatty acids.

Get extra Vitamin C

Vitamin C can lower the amount of histamine found in the blood. Eat lots of fruits and vegetables that contain Vitamin C to ward off any potential problems. It will also help your body fight off any colds.

Monitor pollen & mould counts

If you keep a close eye on the pollen and mold counts, you will know when it is safe to venture outdoors. Keep windows and doors shut to prevent seasonal allergies. However, check the house for mould as well. These can keep your allergies going all year long.

Wash clothes after a visit outdoors during pollen season

The pollen that sets off your seasonal allergies is the microscopic kind. You can't see it, but it gets into your system, which is what drives your body crazy. If you were gardening or went for a walk, take off the clothes you were wearing and wash them as soon as possible. This will help with keeping the pollen at bay.

Wash your hair before bedtime

If you have been outdoors, pollen could be trapped in your hair. What you should avoid is the pollen going from your hair to your pillow and then suffering from seasonal allergies all night long. Wash your hair before going to bed to ensure a good night's sleep.

৷৹৻

WHAT YOU SHOULD KNOW ABOUT SUN ALLERGIES

Sun allergies can be a dangerous reaction to the sun, especially when one does not even know one has it. Sun allergies can resemble sunburn. This is why many people do not even realize that they are allergic to sunlight, commonly called photo-sensitivity.

Here are some things to look for. If you are outside for only a few minutes and already notice redness on the exposed parts of your body, you will have to be careful whenever outdoors. Try to cover up exposed skin by wearing loose fitting clothing, a hat and staying in the shade. Some of the more common places which are affected are the hands, forearms, legs and back of the neck. The rashes could be itchy or burn, and last for a few days. It can go away by itself or you may need to see a doctor. Treatments for sun allergies range from oral beta-carotene to topical creams. The more severe cases can include blisters or hives on the body. You should be especially careful if you develop these symptoms on parts of the body that were clothed, such as the chest and back.

A doctor may perform some more tests such as a biopsy or blood test, to rule out any other problems. There are also medications and lotions that can make the skin more susceptible to sun allergies. Read the label on all products to be safe.

There is a difference between sunburn and sun allergies. Sunburn occurs when the body's protective skin pigment cannot protect the skin well enough from ultraviolet light. When you have an allergy to sunlight, your body's immune system reacts against it. This is what causes the breakout on your skin.

To avoid sun allergies, just a follow a few simple tips:

- ✓ Do not go outside during peak sunlight hours (10 am to 4pm). Your body will have a quicker reaction at this time of day.
- ✓ Do not deliberately sun bathe, even in tanning beds. Those with sun allergies will not be happy with the results.
- ✓ Apply sunscreen 20 minutes before going outdoors. Apply it every two hours after swimming and working out.
- ✓ Dress properly. Wear light clothing, wide-brimmed hats and sunglasses.

Remember, even if you do not suffer from sun allergies, you should always be safe while outdoors. You can get skin cancer and wrinkles from over exposure to the sun. Wear sunscreen and do not stay outside during peak sunlight hours longer than you have to.

ॐ

LAKE WATER ALLERGENS – UNDERSTANDING SWIMMER'S ITCH

Most people cannot resist when they see a nice clear pond or lake. They immediately want to jump or wade into the water. What they do not realize is that there many allergens in the water which can cause serious problems to their skin. Swimming in contaminated water can cause discomforts and skin allergies that can leave scars.

This reaction is known as lake water allergies or swimmer's itch. By contamination it is not meant that they may contain harmful chemical substances which have been released from industries but that which is caused by the animals and birds living around the water body. These birds and animals come to the water bodies to drink water and sometimes even for a swim.

Many of the lakes and ponds carry parasites from birds and animals which are released in to the water especially during summer season when these animals come to the water bodies to drink water. We must understand that the ponds and lakes being the natural habitat of these creatures it is not possible to drive them away and it is up to us humans to stay away from such places and refrain from taking a swim if you are someone prone to allergies.

The symptoms which you can develop if you swim in contaminated water are that your skin begins to burn, itch and start tingling just a few hours after your swim. There are some people whose body will react 12 hours after the swim and develop red pimples all over the body soon after the swim. These nasty pimples can develop into serious blisters if they are not treated quickly. These symptoms will cause plenty of discomfort for a week or so before it actually subsides and can be painful too. Make sure to apply anti allergy creams which will help the blisters to subside and you will be saved from having to go to the hospital.

Some people suffer from more serious problems which can occur due to lake allergies. And this is further aggravated if you continuously expose your body to the contaminated water. Serious symptoms like shortness of breath, fever, nasty skin lesions must be treated immediately and this can cause further complications, so seeing a doctor would be the best thing to do.

৪৩৫৩

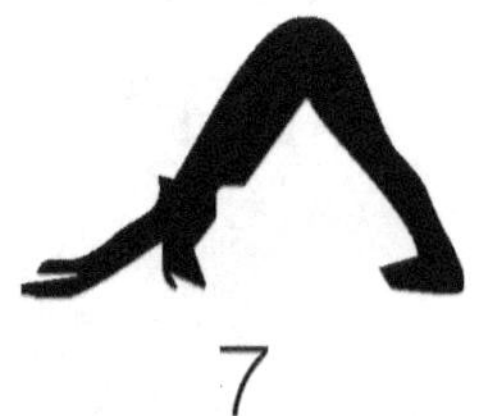

7

MEDICATIONS & ALLERGIES

MEDICATIONS & ALLERGY RELIEF

It is a known fact that 1 in 4 people have allergies. That is a quarter of the world's population. Experts are struggling to find cures rather than palliatives so that people can continue living normal lives.

Different medications can be bought to treat allergies. Your physician will have to prescribe some while others can be purchased over-the-counter. Prescription medicine are used by more than 50% of known allergy patients while 35% take over-the-counter medication.

Oral antihistamines are the most common medications that are prescribed. Most oral antihistamines cause drowsiness and can be bought over-the-counter; there is also the non-drowsy type but it has to be prescribed by a physician. Not all allergy patients obtain the full effect from the non-drowsy types so they go back to the other despite the inconvenience of drowsiness.

Oral antihistamines are not permanent relief – they function on a short term basis only. When taking them, read all the warnings; this medication will react the same way as when one is picked up for OUIL or DUI. The oral treatment can cause drowsiness and keep your brain from thinking and functioning in a normal way. Other side-effects may include anxiety, nausea, loss of appetite, dry mouth and dizziness.

Doctors recommend Benadryl as a temporary quick-fix because of its fast action. It keeps you going till you can get in to see the doctor. Benadryl is a good product to keep in the medicine cabinet for the relief of itching caused from poison ivy and oak, sunburns and insect bites as well as relieving itching from allergies. Use with caution and read the side-effects stated on the label – not everyone can use Benadryl.

Antihistamines can be bought as a nasal spray also when prescribed by the doctor. It increases the concentration where needed and helps to relieve the allergy symptoms at the same time. Using a nasal spray helps to relieve allergy symptoms for up to 12 hours. There are side-effects so be sure to read the warnings. Some of the side-effects are headache and drowsiness. The sprays tend to have a bitter taste as it drips through the nasal passage.

Prescribed medication for the eyes is given for different reasons. Antihistamine drops are for the redness, itching, and swelling in the eyes. Medication for the eyes comes in over-the-counter teardrop form. These drops help to wash out the eyes in order to relieve redness while the antihistamines reduce the itching.

Non-steroidal anti-inflammatory drops are given for the mast cell stabilizer effect to prevent the release of histamine. For chronic symptoms like itching and swelling, Corti-Costeroids drops are given. As for all medications, be sure to consult your physician before using them.

Decongestants come in oral and nasal sprays helping to relieve the allergy symptoms and allowing you to have a better night's sleep. It opens the nasal passages so you are relieved from that stuffy nose feeling. Decongestants can be bought in pill form, sprays and liquids. Like all medications, there are side-effects and warnings so be sure to read the label before using any of them. Doctors advise people who have heart disease, diabetes or are taking certain anti-depressants, not to take decongestion sprays, liquids, etc.

You can find many allergy relief articles and methods on the internet and in books. Do some research and talk to your doctor about getting relief. Learning about herbs can help you find allergy relief too.

Treatments & allergy relief

Recently, studies showed that some of the latest medications and over-the-counter remedies could in fact be responsible for increasing allergies, asthma and other related disease. However, one of the prime medications used to treat asthma proved highly beneficial. The problem was related to the fact that most people who were prescribed these medications over-used the product. This led to more problems.

A bronchodilator, an inhaler which has an Albuterol and Beta-based Agonist medication to treat allergies and asthma, was discovered to bring effective relief to those suffering with these conditions.

The inhaler reopened the airway so that the patient could breathe freely. It quickly resolved mucus build-up. Doctors warned patients against overusing the drug, yet most patients ignored the doctors' warning. They found relief from this medication and used it even when it was not necessary. Now doctors are looking at other remedies to treat allergies and asthma.

How overusing inhalers affects you

Overusing inhalers cause the initial problem to become more severe. In addition, the medication stops doing its thing due to over-use and results in frequent attacks.

How do doctors treat patients now?

Doctors often prescribe Corti-Costeroids. This medication cools inflammation that builds up from infections such as allergies and asthma. Doctors often prescribe Prednisone. This medication has been proven to work, as well as save lives. While this remedy works, it has some dangerous side-effects that showed up adversely in many instances.

How can these medications affect me adversely?

Studies showed that these medications could cause damage to the bones. Glaucoma is affected in some instances. People gained weight while taking this medication, and there were hormonal changes. Dependency was another problem.

The best options

How can one find allergy relief, which does not have adverse effects? You may want to consider yoga. It is a natural workout that teaches one to breathe naturally. Acupuncture also has proven to relieve symptoms stemming from allergies or asthma.

Diet, exercise, yoga and acupuncture may be the best solutions when searching for allergy relief. The natural actions and nutrients will supply the body with what it needs to be healthy. One should also practice avoidance. If one can avoid the irritants, one can find allergy relief.

Products and how they can help you find relief

Dehumidifiers and humidifiers are products that can help you find allergy relief. The filtration systems are designed to purify the air. Some of the impurities that cause asthma and allergy attacks include dust mites, dust, mould, mildew, pollen and so on. These irritants can cause major health problems which are often chronic.

Mould and mildew alone will cause itchy eyes, swelling, rashes, sniffles and so on. Mould and mildew are harsh and should be minimized to avoid allergy attacks and asthma. The products available are designed to purify the air up to 95 percent or higher and remove microns as well as other harmful irritants that cause allergy flare-ups and asthma attacks.

To find allergy relief you should also learn cleaning tips to avoid irritants. Rid your home of dust mites. Dust is something else you must keep down. Mould and mildew cleaners are available but read the labels so that you do not purchase chemicals that cause flare-ups. To learn more about allergy relief go online and read the information available. Do you know what is in the air?

Finding allergy relief with Buster

Today most people have some kind of allergy. Many suffer from hay fever or dust mites allergies – caused by these being present in the carpets and crevices of your home. Dust mites cling to beds and coverings. Doctors suggest medications that do not always work. You may be lucky and they do, but usually, even if they work, the effects do not last long. Your body gets used to it, so it stops being effective, forcing you go to visit the doctor repeatedly. Most medications do not work when people misuse them. Doctors warn patients to avoid over-using medications, yet many fail to listen to the warning in the hope of gaining relief.

All you have to try is this nasal spray made from peppers and a herb called Sting Nettle.

What about this allergy relief?
The name of this allergy relief is called Sinus Buster. It has natural herb ingredients. Sinus Buster has been FDA approved to be safe to take for the relief of allergies. This is made mostly of hot pepper and Stinging Nettle.

you may think that the pepper-based product must sting. According to those who have used it, it does not burn too much. There is some heat which helps get rid of any kind of headache that may occur from allergies. You might want to remember that the more severe the headache, the more heat you will need.

What is in the Sinus Buster?
There is an herb called Stinging Nettle which grows throughout the world. Since it grows plentifully, shortages are unlikely. Although it helps with allergy relief it can cause topical reactions as well if broken and it gets onto the skin. Despite some of its symptoms, these do not last long and normally disappear quickly and quietly.

What can Sinus Buster do for you?
Sinus Buster helps to get instant relief from headaches as well as to breathe better. This Sinus Buster dries and cleans out your nose and sends warmth to your head to take care of that bad headache that comes with allergies. Sinus Buster does not prevent one from getting airborne allergies.

How do you get this wonderful spray?
The best way is to get online and order this spay. It costs $23.99 a bottle in the US.

Concerns
It was discovered that black pepper might be responsible for colon cancer. At present, users of Buster have not reported any adverse effects. Like all medications, you should take this only as recommended by your physician. To learn more about Buster and other new sinus and allergy remedies, go online and check them out.

ॐ

HERBS IN ALLERGY RELIEF

Allergies are a large problem. The dust and pollen quotient in the air gets worse each day.

Herbal based treatments are the all-natural way to stay healthy. Remember when taking herbs, that even though they are considered safe, some of them may counteract your prescribed medications. So, be sure to read and learn about the herbs you are interested in taking to avoid problems. If you do not understand what you are reading, consult your doctor before starting anything new.

Some of the herbs being used today for allergy treatment are Marshmallow root, to help get out mucous from the body; Burdock is used to clear congestion in the respiratory system; to soothe the throat and clear congestion, try using Mullein; to get the antibiotic effect, use Goldenseal Root which contains antibacterial and anti-fungal properties.

Eye Bright is a very effective natural herb to help allergies by combating congestion and hay fever. A natural antihistamine for allergies and fighting infection is Capsicum. Stinging Nettle is used to treat hay fever.

Vitamin C and natural anti-histamine is found in Acerola Cherry. Rosemary is a good anti-inflammatory and strengthens the nervous system too. For reducing mucus and chest congestion, try White Pine.

Using herbs is just one way to help relieve allergy symptoms. Allergies can be deadly to someone with chronic problems. When someone has an allergy attack, they have problems breathing and can begin to hyperventilate as the oxygen level goes down. Remember that herbs are not cures, they only help to relieve the symptoms. Consult a doctor if the symptoms do not seem to go away.

Also important is to keep your home environment as clean as possible from dust, pollen and mould. It could save a life through these mundane precautions.

Dust mites like to live in dark places and where there is moisture. Have a good filter on your sweeper to catch the flying dust before it has a chance to escape. TVs, stereos, furniture and carpets, are just a few of the dust mites' favourite places to multiply. Be sure you clean behind these things and spray the carpets and furniture.

There is also a carpet shampoo to get rid of dust mites imbedded in the carpet and furniture. Keeping the beds free from dust mites is another thing. Encase your box springs, mattress and pillows with a zippered casing.

Check the basement. Mould lives in damp areas and most basements are damp and in need of a dehumidifier. These can be bought at most hardware and department stores. Be sure that it is equipped with a filter on it to keep the dust down along with drawing out the moisture that can cause mould.

₭⌧

www.ingramcontent.com/pod-product-compliance
Lightning Source LLC
Chambersburg PA
CBHW031321250726
48656CB00005B/1910